Willie Tinkle's Search for the Prostate.

Author.------ *David W Eames*

Illustrations.------*Phillip D Eames*

Willie Tinkle's Search for the Prostate.

National Library of Australia
Cataloguing -in-Publication Entry

Eames D.W. (David William)
Willie Tinkle's Search for the Prostate.
1 Prostate-Popular Works. 2. Self-care,Health.1.
Eames.P.D. (Phillip Darren) 11. Title
616. 65

Dedicated to the incredible people who have helped and encouraged me along life's inspirational journey.

Daphne--who filled my life with love and libido.

Our beautiful and caring children
Robyn, Lindsay, and Phillip.

May your smiles bring you life's treasures
And your treasures bring you happy smiles.

Disclaimer

Information provided in this publication is for informational purposes only; it is not intended as a substitute for advice from your own medical team. This information is not to be used for diagnosing or treating any health concerns you may have. Please contact your physician or health care professional for all your medical needs.

Preface

What is a Prostate? The dictionary describes it as, *'gland accessory to the male generative organs in mammals'*. It is a lot more than that.

I would describe its function in the human male as the operator of the grand finale, the cannon fire in the William Tell Overture, the starter's pistol's bang that releases the pent up energy at the start of a marathon race to the human egg.

It nourishes and protects the sperm on its way through a sometimes hostile environment, without the prostate the human race would not exist.

It is like the director of a grand performance, unseen, vital to the end result. On the centre stage 'stands' the star that delivers his performance and then promptly 'hangs' around with his two best friends who happen to live in, well, a sort of a bag.

Wrapped around the urethra it is the gatekeeper of the male urinary system, maybe it tires of the abuse, 22,000 ltrs of urine would pass before it says "Hey, what about me".

It would be expected to contract and expel the seminal fluid on an average of 5,500 times in the average male reproductive life.

We charge headlong along the path of life, savouring its pleasures without so much as a fleeting thought for our sexual health until its too late.

This book has been compiled to help the thousands of men with undiagnosed or unrecognised *Benign Prostate Hyperplasia* (BPH).

This condition is part of the body's warning signs that tells of years of neglect, a poor diet, the lack of exercise that's so important to boost the immune system against attack.

After you read this book you will have informed questions to ask your doctor.

The different medications available, both prescription and natural, advice on surgical procedures when that is your only option.

In the back of the book you will find *Willie Tinkle's Prostate Symptoms Quiz.* Approved by the World Health Organization, (WHO) it can be filled in and presented to your doctor for professional evaluation.

Also in the back is the *Willie Tinkle's Diet to Good Health.* Suitable for both men and women and used in conjunction with the exercise program it will guide the reader to complete general and sexual health lastly, follow Willie Tinkle in his search for the Prostate. I am sure he will bring a smile to your face as he meets the characters along the way.

Introduction

I awoke to the sound of my wife's rhythmic breathing as she slept peacefully by my side.

My mind went back thirty-five years to the days when our children were babies. They would awake in the wee small hours, the slightest whimper, a muffled cough was all it would take and their mother would be out of bed in a flash. She would nourish and comfort them, cradle them in her arms as only a mother knows how, a kiss, a soothing sound as she tucked them back into the cot before she made her way back through the darkened house, getting back into bed as I slept blissfully on.

This is the female of the species, an incredible being, asleep but always in tune for the slightest sound, a sound that will tell her she is needed and will rise to the task without question.

The children have long gone, now I lie in bed awake while my wife sleeps! It has just occurred to me that Mother Nature has played a cruel trick. She has put my bladder in control, is this my punishment for those blissful nights of sleep when the children were little?

Getting out of bed I crept through the cold, darkened house my bladder telling me to hurry, no time to waste! The toilet god accepted my offering and gurgled with pleasure as I crept back to the warm bed, with hands over its face the bedside clock seemed to mock me, 2.10am.

How many times is that to- night, my sleep-deprived brain tried to remember is that two or three, I don't give a bugger, back to sleep.

"Cup of tea dear"? My wife was getting dinner ready as I sat down at the table. "No thanks, I'm cutting back on the fluids, I must be drinking too much tea, I was awake most of the night going to the toilet, no more tea in the afternoon for me".

The summer nights were warm, I tended to be less troubled, and maybe it was just the cold?

During the day the stream was reluctant to start, the flow was brief, and the trips to worship the toilet god were constant.

Shopping trips to unfamiliar territory required checking out the position of facilities as soon as we arrived. "Did you see where the toilets were"? I would say as soon as we entered the shopping center.

I knew the uncontrollable urge that I had become familiar with would rear its head at awkward moments, like going through the checkouts!

We have a saying in Australia "siphon your python". Well, my python wouldn't siphon and as I stood in the corner embarrassed, people came and went, at last my turn came in the form of a weak dribble. I felt the job was only half done, this proved to be the case in later tests.

As my symptoms progressed I decided to make an appointment with my local GP. He suggested that I had an enlarged prostate and ordered a blood test.

The PSA reading came back at 4.5. He booked an appointment for a DRE (Digital Rectal Examination), "Your prostate gland is enlarged but I can't feel any lumps so that's good news. A lump may indicate the presence of cancer. I suggest we adopt the "Watch and Wait" technique to see if theres any change".

I was sitting in the doctor's office not knowing what to say, I didn't know anything about this condition, the questions to ask, the treatment available. Rising from my seat I thanked the doctor and left, my first big mistake.

The years past, I learned to suffer the multiple night trips to the toilet. Public facilities meant a change of tactics. Instead of using the urinal and suffer the embarrassment of the dreaded dribble, I used the cubical where I could hide my self imposed shame.

Visiting relatives and friends with overnight stays provided another set of problems.

Creeping around an unfamiliar house in the middle of the night, the creaking floorboards, trying to remember where the furniture was placed in the pitch black darkness, tripping over the toys, silently cursing as I made my way to worship the toilet god. Pushing the button would be met with a seemingly deafening roar as the water rushed into the cistern, I would imagine the whole household being awakened as I crept sheepishly back to my bed.

One morning when I went there was a burning as I passed water, the urine looked cloudy instead of the normal colour, my system was telling me it couldn't go on any longer.

"You have a bladder infection; I will give you a course of antibiotics that should clear this up". I watched the doctor write out a prescription, aware of a dull ache in my pelvic area, my lower back was tender. Did I hurt it lifting something?

The following week was hell, my Willie felt like someone had shoved a red-hot poker up the middle, the urine didn't look good at all, and in fact it looked disgusting.

The day that I couldn't pee at all my desperation became obvious. Constant tries resulted in a few drops yellow liquid.

Lying on my back in a female doctor's surgery, bare from the waist down, was not my favourite pass-time. She pressed gently on my distended lower abdomen. "You have acute urine retention; we will have to insert a catheter into the penis to drain your bladder".

I nodded in approval as she disappeared through the surgery door returning with the attending nurse in tow.

I watched as the nurse removed the folley catheter from its sterile wrapping, and with gloved hands injected an anesthetic lubricant into the tip of my Willie. Holding Willie in one hand she inserted the catheter with the other, the collection bag already hanging on the side of the surgery bed.

The relief was instant; I was on my way to having the relief I had sought for 15 long years.

The nurse flitted in and out of the room checking on my progress, looking at the bag. "You're doing well – she said encouragingly, seven hundred and fifty mills already".

One and a half litres of urine were drained that day; I was amazed that the bladder could hold all that without bursting. I left the surgery with a collection bag attached and went home.

The first night I lay on my side with the drain tube from my Willie over the side of the bed and into the collection bag at the side. That was the best night's sleep that I had for many years, no getting up to go to the toilet, I felt relaxed, the burning had lessened although the infection was still present.

My referral was to attend the outpatient section of the nearest hospital "We are going to remove the catheter then the doctor will see you". The attending casualty nurse was deflating the balloon that held it in place.

I watched as she pulled it out, a small amount of blood was evident. "You can go back to the waiting room and take a seat; a doctor will see you as soon as one is available".

He seemed tired as he looked over my admission file. The dark complexion tended to hide the shadowy circles forming under his lower eyelids, his voice was dull, lifeless, almost uninterested.

"I am going to give you a medication called Mini-Pres, it works by relaxing the muscles at the bladder neck and the sphincter, and it should improve your voiding". I stood up and turned toward the door.

"Oh by the way, take them before you retire at night they tend to make some patients dizzy".

The Mini-Pres didn't work, I was back to square one, and the infection wasn't getting any better I had to get an appointment with the Urologist as soon as possible.

By this time, I had watched the nurses inserting the catheter, it was a very simple process, and the main requirement was to follow a strict hygiene routine.

I was in trouble, the weekend was upon me, and in desperation I decided to make my own makeshift catheter! The relief was instant, used twice a day and before going to bed I at last had complete control over my renegade bladder.

I had bought myself time – the time needed to enable me to get an appointment with the urologist.

At last my appointment time came, a smile spread across the doctor's face as I revealed my desperation, the homemade in and out catheter.

"I think we can do a bit better than that, he smiled, I will ask the nurse to get you a real one".

He reached for the computer keyboard and started to type. "This is a special anti-biotic that will clear up the bladder infection, in the meantime I will book you in for an operation which will clear the obstruction caused by your enlarged prostate gland".

I looked after that clear plastic Nelaton FG12 catheter like it was made of precious metal, the infection cleared completely, I was ready for the operation.

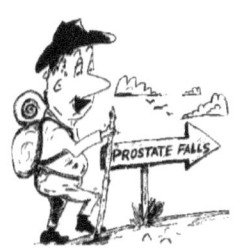

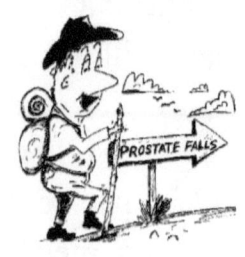

Secret Men's Business

Table of Contents.

Page #

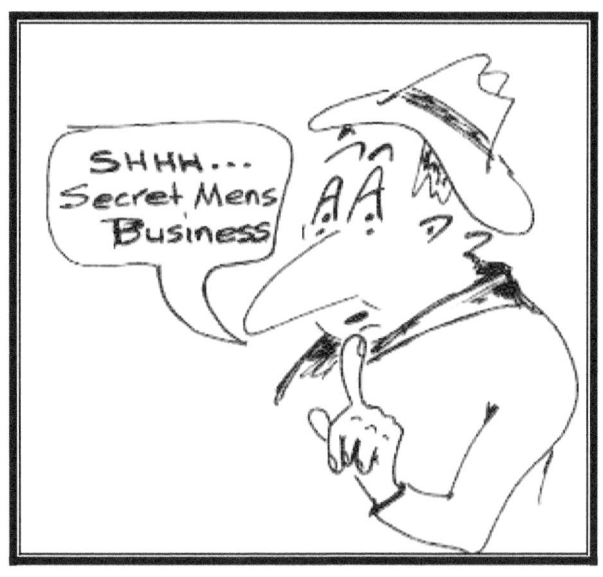

Chapter 1

Men's secret disease.

It begins so gradually and imperceptibly that you may not even notice it. You visit the rest rooms several more times than usual during the day – maybe you're just drinking more water. You interrupt business meetings for a bathroom break a lot more often than your friends and work mates. You haven't sat through an entire concert or movie for years, and when you fly you always ask for an aisle seat so as not to disturb fellow passengers with your frequent trips to the toilet. It's slightly annoying and more than a bit embarrassing, but not a cause for major concern. Or so you think.

At night, though, you begin to realise that something has changed. Your sleep is interrupted by toilet calls as often as every two to three hours. Being awakened four times a night and feeling lousy every day because of the sleep deprivation – does make you a bit worried and confused. Maybe it is stress, your diet or those beers in the afternoon after work?

Looking for a medical answer, you may attribute your difficulties to a shrinking bladder, but in fact this condition has nothing to do with your bladder. This *increased frequency of the need to urinate* is probably the first noticeable and major sign of a growing prostate, *benign prostatic hyperplasia* (BPH), more commonly referred to by the public as an *"enlarged prostate"* (hyperplasia means "an enlargement due to an increased number of cells") BPH. Is a secret, silent disease. Silent because men commonly don't feel its progression and secret because men who have it – most will during their lifetime – don't talk about it.

It's so prevalent that comedians frequently joke about the symptoms ("a good night is one in which you only have to get up once"). The symptoms run the gamut from merely annoying, to downright uncomfortable, to in the worst scenario, totally excruciating.

Benign prostatic hyperplasia is the most common noncancerous (benign means "non-malignant") tumour in men and ranks with prostate cancer as the two most common prostate disorders affecting middle-aged and older men.

What we know (from autopsy studies of men who died from causes other than prostate enlargement) is that a man's prostate typically starts to enlarge at about age 45, although about 10 per cent of men between the ages of 25 to 30 years also have BPH. By age 50, about half of all men will have some noticeable signs of the disease. The number rises to 60 per cent at age 60 and continues to escalate over the next two and a half decades, until by the time they reach 85 years of age, 90 per cent of all men suffer significant symptoms. In other words, if they live long enough, nearly all men will develop microscopic evidence of BPH.

The condition does not seem to be related to sexual activity or lack thereof, since it occurs in celibate priests with the same frequency as sexually active men and is also not related to either sexual excesses or deprivation.

Although BPH may be inevitable for most men, the annoying symptoms don't have to be. At no time in history have so many good treatment options been available, and never before have so many men actively sought out these options.

David Eames

Hyperplasia, what is that?
Does it stand for a Willie that's flat?
No---it doesn't stand for that at all
Read this chapter and you will see
It stands for a Willie that cannot pee

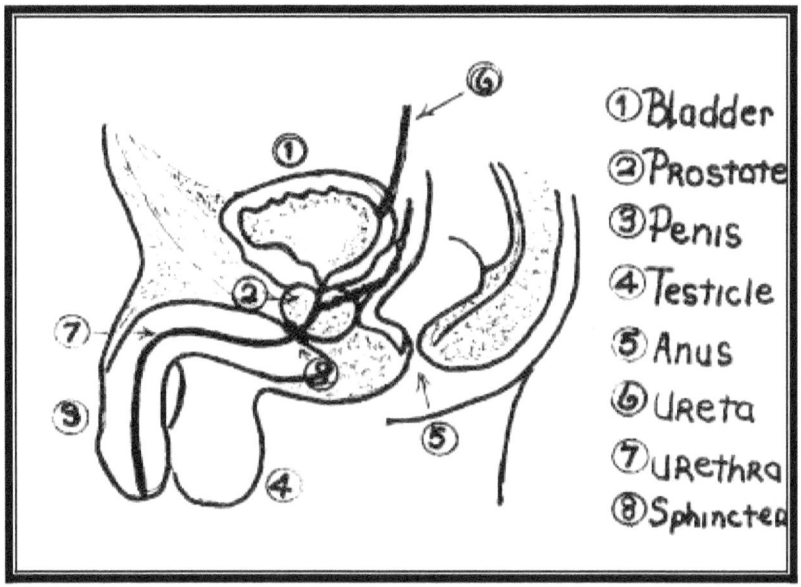

1. Bladder
2. Prostate
3. Penis
4. Testicle
5. Anus
6. Ureta
7. Urethra
8. Sphincter

Chapter 2

The Prostate Gland

When a baby is born the prostate is about the size of a pea, and it thereafter grows slowly until reaching almond-size at the onset of puberty. Under the influence of sex hormones, the prostate then begins a stage of more rapid continual growth until a man reaches his late 20's or early 30's, by which time it is about the size of a walnut or large chestnut and weighs a little less than an ounce. Partly glandular and partly composed of smooth muscle tissue the prostate surrounds the neck of the bladder and wraps around the urethra (the thin tube leading from the bladder through the penis, and through which both urine and sperm pass from the body).

Because the prostate is only indirectly involved in procreation, it is considered an accessory rather than a key part of the male reproductive system, but it nevertheless is a particularly vulnerable part of the male anatomy. To help visualise this, think of the prostate as a fist holding a straw (the urethra).

Beginning somewhere around 40 cells in most men's prostate commence to multiply again, and they continue to do so slowly until death. The enlarged tissue of the prostate is like the fist squeezing the straw, thereby making it difficult for urine too pass through the urethra.

In severe cases the prostate can grow up to 10 times its normal size. In relatively few men, the prostate actually shrinks or atrophies during later years. Although many small glands within the prostate secrete several different substances, we know now that its key function is to produce and discharge the viscid, alkaline fluid that comprises a major portion of the seminal fluid.

The prostatic fluid helps to maintain an appropriate environment, in which sperm can live; provides them with some nourishment; and in general increases their survival time after ejaculation.

The prostatic fluid also contains prostaglandins, a hormone like fatty acid that effect smooth muscle fibres and blood vessel walls.

One of the many theories about the prostaglandin's produced by the prostate is that they encourage the cervix (the entrance to the female uterus) to dilate, thus enabling the sperm to pass through it and fertilise the egg.

During ejaculation, the muscles in the prostate contract, pushing the fluid through special ducts into the urethra, however the prostate is never totally emptied. Sperm, produced in the testes, also enter the urethra via a tube called the vas deferens. With ejaculation the sperm, prostatic fluid and other fluids combine to carry the sperm out of the body.

The part of the prostate that surrounds the urethra is considered the middle lobe and is sometimes called the central zone. It is enveloped by larger, peripheral zones on either side of the urethra. These zones are composed primarily (about 75 per cent) of glands, which are usually the primary sites where cancer develops, although cancer of the peripheral ducts can arise in the central zone. A small transitional zone lies within the middle lobe, adjacent to the urethra sphincter and *is the sole site of benign prostatic hyperplasia.*

Before enlargement, this small transition zone comprises only 2 per cent of the entire mass of a normal prostate gland.

As the tissue in the transitional zone grows, true prostate tissue is displaced and the prostate gland gradually becomes grossly enlarged. The new growth is composed of the same general type of tissue as the normal prostate except that it is more fibrous and muscular in nature. The growth typically occurs in an asymmetrical manner, extending most of the way or part of the way around the prostatic urethra (that part of the urethra surrounded by the prostate) and begins to constrict the urethra.

The effects of the BPH on the urethra can vary, depending on the nature of the growth. If it enlarges in a primary outward direction, for example the prostate can reach a huge size, relatively speaking yet not cause any significant obstructive symptoms of the urethra. Some men with greatly enlarged prostates experience little or no obstruction whereas some relatively small prostates produce severe obstruction.

The prostate plays no direct role in the functioning of the male's urinary system, but because it is situated close to the bladder and the urethra, a myriad of urinary problems can result. In fact, BPH symptoms occur primarily because enlargement of the prostate constricts the urethra and obstructs urinary flow. Prostatic infection also can result in painful or burning sensation.

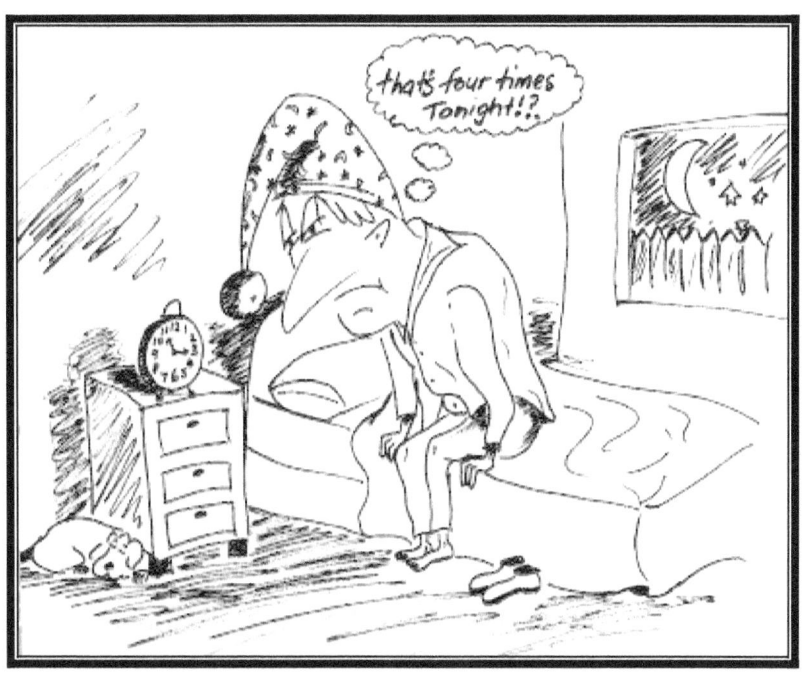

Chapter 3

The Symptoms of BPH.

Nocturia.

The number of times that men are awakened during the night varies with the degree of urinary obstruction, however, in severe cases, it may occur hourly. The fatigue that results from frequent awakening during the night is only one of the side effects of obstructive symptoms of BPH.

Frequency.

The feeling of needing to urinate even after having done so is a second major symptom of BPH. Only minutes after urinating you may experience the sensation that your bladder is not empty and that you need to urinate again. This symptom is one of the most distressing results of BPH. This occurs because of the enlarging prostate pushes on the bottom of the bladder and reduces its capacity to hold urine; hence the increased frequency and the signalling of a false need for urination.

Another related cause is that *residual urine from a not-completely-emptied bladder* reduces the bladders functional capacity. Think of a four litre container that is never less than half-full and must be emptied twice as often, having a capacity now of only two litres. The retention of the urine in the bladder can also cause enlargement and loss of ability to contract.

Straining or hesitancy.

Many men with BPH experience difficulty in starting urination. Author Michael Korda describes it as one of the "better-known humiliations of the ageing process in men".

You may be busy, travelling, or occupied with the job you may be doing at the time and delay the need to urinate, especially if the need to urinate occurs with great frequency.

If you hold it for more than a few minutes after the first urge however, you may experience an involuntary burst of urine. More commonly your entire urinary system may seem to *"close down"*, and you may barely be able to start a urinary stream. This delay is called *"hesitancy"*.

When this happens, you may spend what seems like endless minutes standing at the toilet, pushing and straining to force the urine out and sometimes having to repeat the process several times until a normal flow is regained. During this time you may have a urinary stream that barely dribbles despite the sense that the bladder is full. Why hesitancy occurs is not clear, but it may be due to the time it takes to attain sufficient pressure within the bladder to overcome the resistance caused by the obstructing prostate.

In extreme cases of difficulty with urination – what the medical world calls *"acute complete urinary retention"* you may have to go to hospital for emergency catheterization. This is rare and is unlikely to occur unexpectedly, but when it does happen it is a painful and emotionally disturbing situation.

Intermittency.

Another common symptom of BPH is *dribbling at the end of urination.* Doctor's call this *"intermittency"* but you may know it more intimately as that embarrassing dark spot on your trousers that appears uncontrollably after you have zipped up.

It occurs because as the prostatic obstruction grows, the bladder can't empty completely with a single muscle contraction. Seconds later however the muscle involuntarily contracts a second time and a small stream of urine – raging from a few drops to 20mls or more escapes.

Taken together these common symptoms of BPH are called *prostatism.* Although BPH is their most frequent cause, other disorders, such as prostate or bladder infections can also produce the same collection of symptoms. At their worst, these symptoms may signal prostate cancer. But remember

BPH *is not prostate cancer, and having it doesn't mean that you are any more likely to get prostate cancer than someone who is not so affected.*

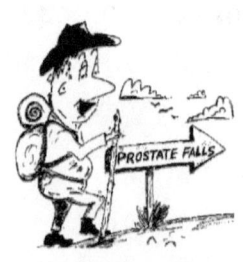

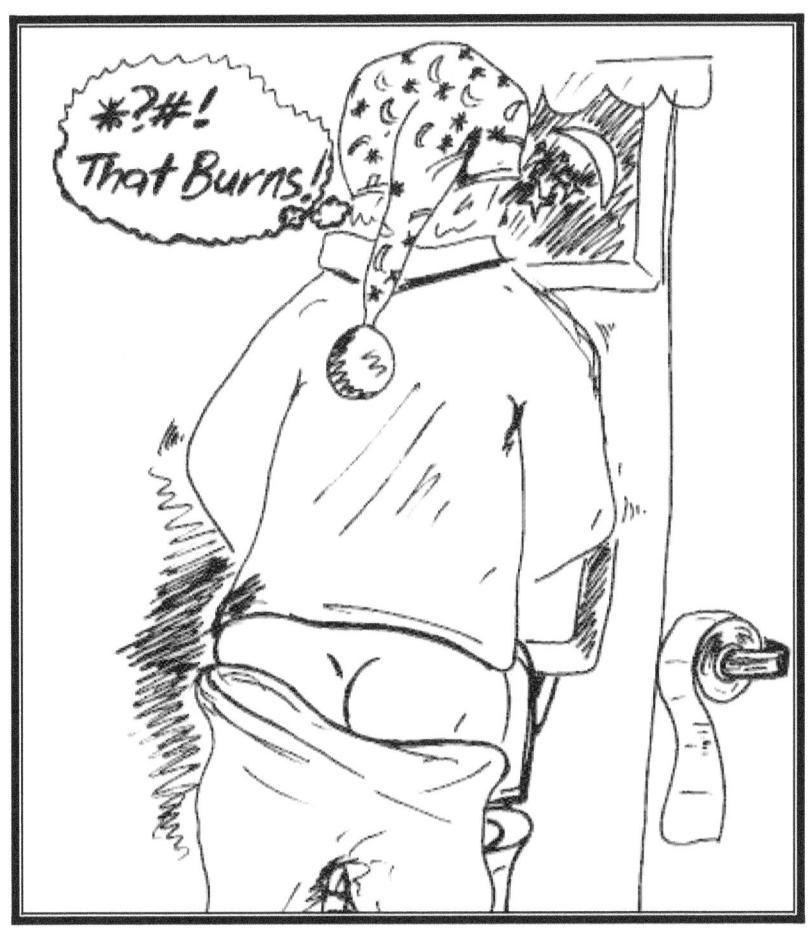

Chapter 4

Long Range Effects of BPH.

Where BPH frequently results in incomplete urine elimination it can lead to bladder infections and cystitis (inflammation), with unpleasant symptoms that range from burning during urination to constant severe pain. While these side affects of BPH are curable with antibiotics, they are likely to recur frequently, creating another costly, inconvenient and pain filled experience. Because stagnant urine is an almost ideal fluid for nurturing the growth of bacteria, *incomplete bladder emptying* causes a circular effect in which the bladder's inability to discharge urine called *"stasis"* predisposes the upper urinary and bladder to *infections.*

Inflammation from these infections can lead to tissue changes, usually thickening of the tissue, which is considered by some as the cause of many of the more bothersome symptoms of BPH. Bacteria growing in the urine tend to make it highly alkaline, which can also lead to the formation of *stones in the bladder* with once again severe pain and discomfort. Since they tend to gravitate towards the neck of the bladder, the stones may sometimes cause an obstruction there. They can also pass through the neck of the bladder and become lodged in the urethra, and if they continue to pass through, cause *extreme pain* with their passage.

When the bladder has to work harder and contract more forcefully to expel urine, its inner surface becomes thick and irregular a condition known as *"trabeculation"*. This irregular thickening leaves areas of weakness in the lining of the bladder, which may extend outward to form small pouches, called *"deverticula"*. These pockets may not drain properly, causing stones to form within them. At its extreme, BPH can lead to *incontinence,* where a man no longer has control over his bladder's functioning. He may not even be able to sense when he is urinating, making the wearing of adult pads an uncomfortable and often embarrassing necessity. Sustained or prolonged obstruction due to BPH can result in more severe conditions such as development of kidney stones, as well as *bladder and kidney damage,* which in turn may result in life threatening *renal failure* and excess of urea in the blood.

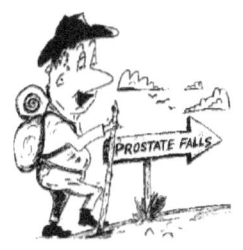

The Prostate is a gland you see
Its home is sometimes a mystery
Around the Urethra and under the Bladder
Lives two nuts in a bag---Joe and Adder.

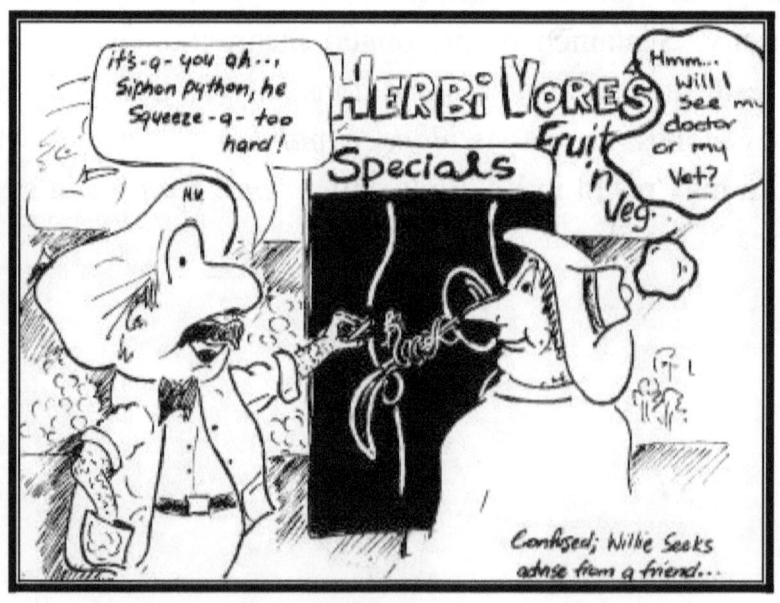

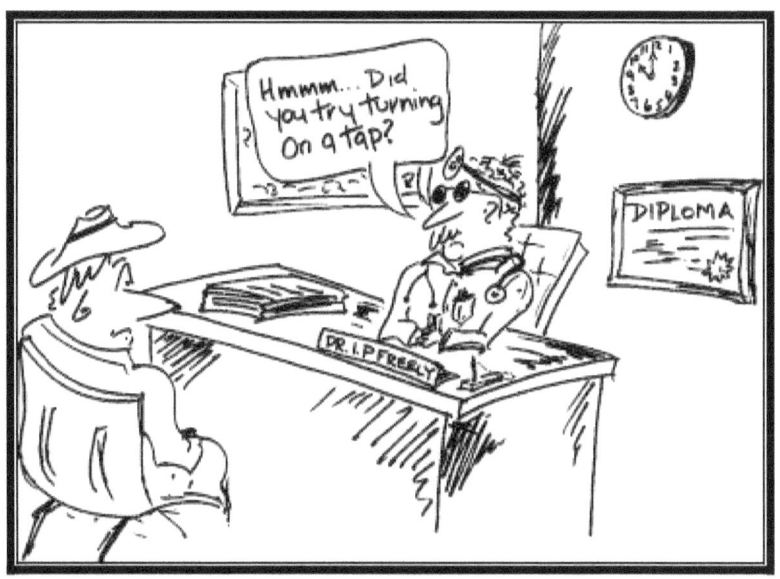

Chapter 5

Consulting Your Doctor.

The obvious and painful symptoms discussed in the proceeding paragraphs generally become progressively more difficult to ignore. If you are experiencing some or all of them, their presence may indicate that you have BPH. To rule out prostate cancer or other prostate problems, you should undergo testing which will confirm BPH.

One common test is the *digital rectal exam* (DRE) which involves the doctor inserting a lubricated-gloved finger up your rectum to the point where he can feel the prostate gland through the wall of the rectum. A normal prostate feels smooth and elastic, while an enlarged prostate may feel rubbery. Size can be misleading; however, as a prostate that is small by rectal examination can still be sufficiently enlarged to cause obstruction. Treatment options for BPH depend, of course not on size but on the severity of the disease for the man involved.

Another test the doctor may order is an examination of a *urine specimen.* Although the *urinalysis* does not directly contribute to the diagnosis of BPH it helps the doctor rule out urinary tract infections (shown by the presence of a large number of white blood cells or by bacteria) and look for blood in the urine, which may indicate BPH, but can also warn of kidney or bladder disease.

A blood test will help rule out other disorders and typically include a determination of PSA (*prostate specific antigen)* and *alkaline phosphatase levels* to screen for cancer. A *serum creatinine measurement* to determine whether or not there are kidney complications. Other diagnostic procedures might include urodynamic measurement of *urine flow and bladder pressure* to help determine the degree of obstruction, the functioning of the bladder and urinary sphincters.

The doctor may also recommend a *cystoscopy,* an uncomfortable procedure in which he inserts a tube that contains a lens and a light system through the opening of the urethra after a solution is sent into the urethra that numbs the inside of the penis. With the cystoscope the doctor can determine the size of the prostate gland and identify the location and degree of the obstruction of the urethra. The cystoscope exam can also give an accurate measurement of the amount of residual urine in the bladder if the doctor has had the patient urinate immediately prior to the examination. As the cystoscope enters the bladder any urine that remains inside comes out of the cystoscope and can be collected and measured.

The more residual urine (especially if it *exceeds 100mls)* the greater the need for surgical treatment.

Fortunately, all of the diagnostic procedures discussed in the proceeding paragraphs can be carried out on an outpatient basis.

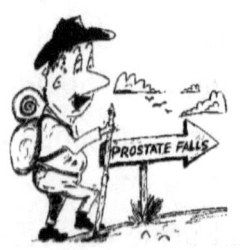

Chapter 6

Treating BPH.

Evaluation of the treatment options for men with BPH include considering not only the severity of the symptoms, although that may be the reason to consult with your doctor, but also the type of treatment to suit the patient. This in turn is influenced by the risk entailed; the advantages/disadvantages in any procedure or medication chosen, and the health related quality of life with or without treatment.

Both direct considerations (cost of diagnosis, management, treatment and post treatment monitoring) and indirect consideration (loss of work time, negative impact on well being) should also be taken into account. Sometimes the existence of other health problems will necessarily influence the decision.

Although there are several medical options that are under investigation, and more will be undoubtedly introduced over the next decade, at present there are three major ways BPH is treated.

Watchful Waiting.

From a physician's viewpoint, watchful waiting (as its name implies) means no active treatment, but periodic examinations to evaluate progression of BPH. Is it appropriate for many men, particularly those who are asymptomatic or have only mild symptoms, and whose enlarged prostate was likely found through the digital rectal examination.

The natural history of untreated BPH is poorly documented in literature. Both the severity of obstruction can fluctuate considerably over time. Some studies have shown that a significant proportion of men with moderate BPH symptoms (between 50 and 75 per cent) experienced either stabilisation or improvement of their symptoms in the absence of any therapeutic intervention.

More recent studies show that 30 per cent of men with BPH will experience little or no change in symptoms with watchful waiting. For unknown reasons, a small number (about 15 per cent) actually improve over time, however, some 56 per cent of men are likely to experience a worsening of symptoms.

Certainly it appears that the decision to select *watchful waiting* as a "treatment" choice depends not only on the physical evaluation of a man's symptoms and his restriction in activities, but also on the *quality-of-life* considerations such as discomfort level and lifestyle restrictions, and how worrisome the condition is for the man involved.

Transurethral Resection of the Prostate (TURP).

The "gold standard" against which all other treatments for BPH are measured is transurethral resection of the prostate, commonly referred to as TURP, and more flippantly, some doctors refer to this operation as a "rebore". Although TURP has been the surgical treatment of choice for BPH for the past 50 years, and the one against which all newer techniques are compared, 20 per cent of patient's experience clinically significant adverse reactions following surgery, and between 5 per cent and 15 percent require a second operation after two years of follow up.

TURP involves removing those portions of the prostate that are obstructing the urethra by inserting an instrument called a *resectoscope* through the urethra into the bladder. It uses a telescopic hot wire loop that emits a high-frequency electrical current to cut like an electric knife through the prostate gland, working outward until the surgical capsule is reached. The pieces of tissue that are cut away, called "chips" are carried by irrigating fluid into the bladder and then flushed out through the resectoscope. Samples of tissue are sent to the laboratory to be examined for prostate cancer.

TURP is the operation of choice for small and moderate growth of BPH, but not for patients with massive BPH, since it is technically difficult to do in such cases.

TURP is major surgery. Although no incision is made, general or spinal anaesthesia is required. It is a delicate procedure, requires a skilled surgeon, and can take anywhere from 30 to 90 minutes to complete. Hospitalisation lasts from two to five days, (a tube or catheter is inserted in the bladder for the first two or three days) after which a man can expect to spend two to four weeks at home recovering. Significant side effects associated with TURP include *temporary bleeding,* the chance of urinary or other *infections* (as with any surgery), *retrograde ejaculation* (semen passing into the bladder on ejaculation) occurring in 70 to 75 per cent of patients. *Temporary urinary retention* after the removal of the catheter, *impotence* (occurring in 5 to 10 per cent of cases) and *incontinence* (in about 2 to 4 per cent of cases), not to mention cardiac risk due to anaesthesia. In addition, anywhere from 2 to 10 percent of patients require blood transfusions. Late postoperative complications include urethral stricture (abnormal narrowing or constriction) and contractures of the bladder neck.

Medical studies differ with regard to exact statistics on impotence caused by surgery, because many men may be impotent and undiagnosed before TURP is performed. In a review of literature, Dr. Taivo Tammela, an urologist associated with Tampere University Hospital in Tampere, Finland cited a 1995 study that suggested that there were *virtually no new cases of impotence or incontinence after TURP.*

The symptoms of a renegade gland
Are two weary eyes and a reason to stand
The call of the toilet ---Willie in hand
A job not yet finished---try again soon
Give Willie a shake and feel like a Goon.

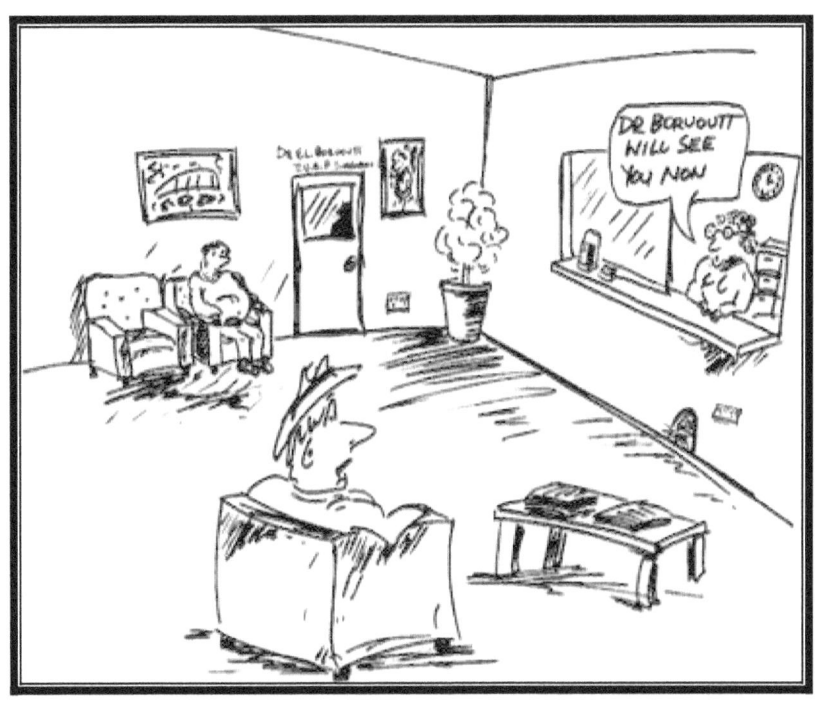

David Eames

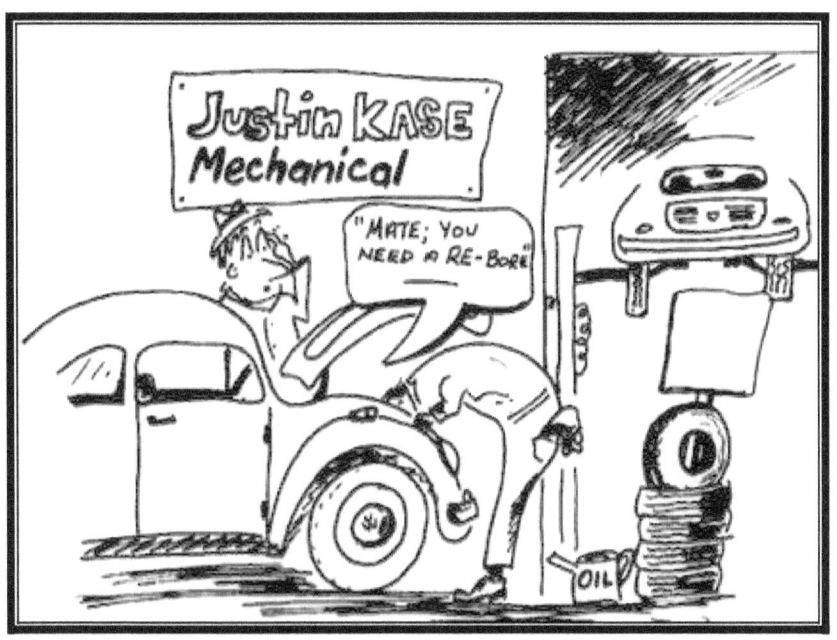

Chapter7

The TURP Operation.

Consent and risks.

Consent is a legal document recognising your willingness to proceed with the intended treatment. You are required to *sign a consent form* for the operation once you fully understand the reason for the operation and the risks involved.

All operations have risks associated with them. The risks should be discussed with your doctor. You should understand the procedure and any available *alternative treatment.* Your local doctor may also be able to answer your questions.

Preadmission.

Preadmission is the assessment you have before your operation. You will attend a clinic in your local hospital. This assessment will usually be taken about a week prior to your admittance for the operation. There are numerous tests that may be required for your preadmission such as:

EGC (a tracing of your heart)
Chest x-ray
Urine test
Blood test
Height and weight

Blood pressure/pulse and temperature

Other test may be necessary if you have diabetes, asthma or heart problems etc. You will be interviewed by a number of people.

A doctor will explain your operation, obtain your consent and answer any questions you have.

Prepare yourself and write down any questions you may have, and please, don't be afraid to ask.

An anaesthetist will explain their role during your operation and will discuss pain relief after the surgery. They will also assess your general health.

A Pharmacist may see you to discuss your prescribed medication and any changes that may be needed.

Nursing staff will also discuss your operation with you. They will outline what to expect before and after surgery, and will answer any questions you may have.

Discharge Preparation.

The usual length of stay for your TURP operation is 3 days. You should plan your transport home, as this is not provided by the hospital (unless an ambulance is needed for medical reasons). When arranging transport, please be aware that you should not drive for 24hrs after anaesthetic. Your family should be aware that you would also need some assistance with household chores during the first few weeks after discharge.

Your medication.

Some medications *can increase the risk of bleeding from surgery.* Most of these medications are used for pain relief. Please discuss your medication with your doctor, as some may need to be stopped for 1-2 weeks before your procedure.

At your preadmission interview with your doctor take along a list of any medication that you may be using to allow him to assess them. Some medications are taken for *blood clotting.* These are usually prescribed for people who have developed clots in blood vessels or lungs in the past e.g.

Warfarin, Marevan, Dindevan

Let your doctor know if you are taking any of these medications well before your procedure.

The following medications may be taken as alternatives for pain relief.

Paracetamol, Panadol, Panamax, Panadiene,Panadiene Forte.

What to bring to the Hospital.

All medications and x-rays.
Pyjamas / dressing gown.
Comfortable shoes or slippers.
Toiletries and tissues.
Reading material.
Medicare / healthcare cards.

Wedding rings may be worn; however other *jewellery and valuables should be left at home.*

Bring only *enough cash to meet travel needs and other short stay requirements.*

The Day of the Operation.

You will be going to the theatre from Pre-Surgery Ward or if an inpatient from the Urology Ward. In the morning you will require another shower with an antiseptic soap. You will also be supplied with theatre clothes to change into.

Your anaesthetist may prescribe a premedication for you to have before you go to the theatre. This may be an injection or a tablet, which helps to prepare your anaesthetic. It may give you a dry mouth or make you feel drowsy. After having the premedication, you may also be unsteady on your feet so you should remain in bed until a nurse assists you onto the theatre trolley. On arrival in theatre you will be introduced to the theatre staff who will ask you some questions to confirm your identity and the operation you are to have.

After the Operation.

After your operation you will be transferred to the recovery room where you will be monitored until you are awake. You will then be escorted back to the ward.

After the operation you may have the following

An IV tube drip in your arm for hydration.

An oxygen mask is sometimes worn the first few hours to assist with your breathing. A fine tube called a *catheter* will have been inserted into your bladder to drain the urine. This is connected to *"bladder washout bags" (irrigation's)*. These gently irrigate the bladder and prevent the formation of blood clots, which may block the catheter.

A nurse will monitor your temperature, pulse, blood pressure and irrigation's. This will continue on a regular basis and sometimes throughout the night.

Your nurse will ask you if you have pain. Pain relief is very important to your recovery. Please do not be afraid to ask for more pain relief.

On return to the ward you will need to rest in bed for 4hrs. You can eat and drink after this period. A nurse will provide assistance with your catheter bag when you walk if necessary.

For good circulation, leg exercises, deep breathing and change of position is encouraged while you are resting in bed.

While the catheter is present it may stimulate the inside of your bladder giving you the feeling it is full or it may cause a spasm where urine may leak outside of the catheter. Please tell your nurse if these problems occur.

Your catheter will be checked for blockages. Spasms, although uncomfortable, are usually harmless and should settle once the catheter is removed.

The Next Two Days

The wash out bags connected to your catheter will be removed the morning following your surgery. Drink a glass of water every hour to "flush" blood out of your bladder.

Your catheter will be removed Day 2 after your surgery. *Stinging and burning may occur when passing urine for 1 or 2 days.* Increasing your fluid intake and taking a medicated powered drink such as Citralite or Ural available from the nurse can relieve this.

Your drinking and voiding will be measured and documented. If your voiding pattern is satisfactory you may be discharged home in the afternoon.

Home Advice-Activity.

Avoid straining and heavy lifting for six weeks after the operation. Walking is the best form of exercise. After one week slowly increase the distance you walk each day.

You should not drive for 1-2 weeks after the operation, riding a bicycle should be avoided.

Drinking. Drink 2-3 litres of fluid a day to flush out the blood from your urine. This may continue for 3 weeks after the operation.

Bowels. It is important to keep your bowels soft and regular to avoid straining. Bran, exercise and drinking plenty of water should ensure this.

Bleeding.

The surgery leaves a raw area on the inside of the prostate. This will form a scab as it heals. You will pass some of this scab in your urine for up to one month.If this occurs with bleeding it is suggested you limit your activity and increase fluids further until the bleeding settles down.

Continence.

Although patients generally experience some difficulties with urine control following the removal of the catheter, most have excellent control when they leave the hospital. However, a few may experience episodes of incontinence, which may need treatment with medication, pelvic muscle exercises or other.If you are experiencing problems report them to your treating doctor.

Sexual Function.

Following prostatic surgery, when ejaculation occurs, the semen does not come out immediately through the penis. Instead it passes into the bladder and is passed out with the urine. This is due to the bladder neck being removed with the prostate. Because of this, most men will be sterile; however, normal contraceptive measures should be maintained as some semen may leak.

Although ejaculation does not occur, a normal orgasm is still experienced. The operation does not usually affect the ability to obtain an erection. Refrain from sexual activity until advised by your doctor.

In Case of Problems.

If you develop any of the following:
Inability to pass urine.
Dark blood stained urine. (Especially blood clots)
Fevers, chills, sweats.
Worsening discomfort when passing urine.
Contact your urology unit, your doctor or the emergency department of your hospital.

David Eames

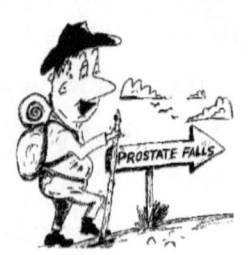

If your Willie won't pee---you'll regret it, you see
Stones in the bladder---a burning like fire
Your Willie will burn--- like a second hand tyre
Hell---you may even lose all your sexual desire!

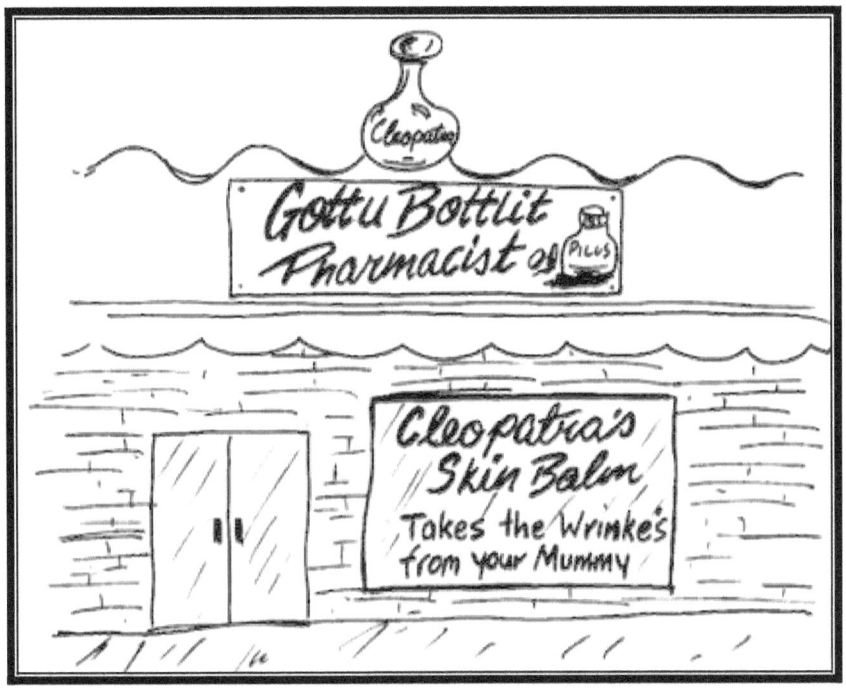

Chapter 8

Medication

Alpha-Advenergic Blockers

Hytrin is the brand name of a systemic drug called *teragosin* (ter- AY-zoe-sin) which has been used to treat high blood pressure since 1987.

The Food and Drug Administration (FDA) approved its use to treat BPH in 1993.

Hytrin is a long-acting, highly selective alpha-advenergic blocking agent. *It works by relaxing the smooth muscles in the prostate and the opening of the bladder.* For many men, the urinary channel passage then opens enough to increase the flow of urine and also to decrease such symptoms as the need to urinate and a weak stream. In no way does it help shrink the prostate, which may continue to grow resulting ultimately in the symptoms becoming worse over time. So even though Hytrin may lesson some of the symptoms over a period of time as long as six weeks, surgery may still be needed in the future.

Hytrin's most common side effects are *dizziness* or *vertigo* due to the *lowering of the patient's blood pressure.* It occurs in 7.2 to 15.6 per cent of patients. Some physicians recommend that the dose be taken in the evening or at bedtime to avoid the dizziness that occurs upon standing (called postural hypertension) and other blood pressure related side effects, however it has been shown that morning administration is well tolerated by some patients.

Other side effects can include *chest pain, light-headedness* when rising from a lying or sitting position (1.9 to 3.9 per cent of patients) *sudden fainting, weakness, fatigue and drowsiness* (3.6 to 8.0 per cent) *a fast, irregular or pounding heart beat* (0.9 to 1.6 per cent) *shortness of breath, nasal congestion, swelling of the feet and lower legs, and impotence* (1.0 to 1.6 per cent of patients).

Other alpha-advenergic blockers that work on the same principle as Hytrin include *Cardura* (doxazosin) with side effects of dizziness, drowsiness and headaches, and shorter acting drugs such as *Minipress* (prazosin) and *Xatral* (alfuzosin). Minipress must be taken two to three times a day and may, like Cardura cause dizziness and headaches.

In contrast to other alpha-blockers, *Tamsulosin* brand name *Flomax,* which need to be taken only once daily, has no significant effect on blood pressure.

It is available in a modified release formulation, which enables men to take it once daily.

In an American study, the adverse side affects that accured with Tamsulosin than with a placebo were *abnormal ejaculation and rhinitis* (inflammation of the mucus membranes of the nose).

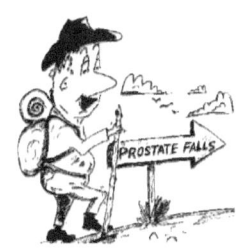

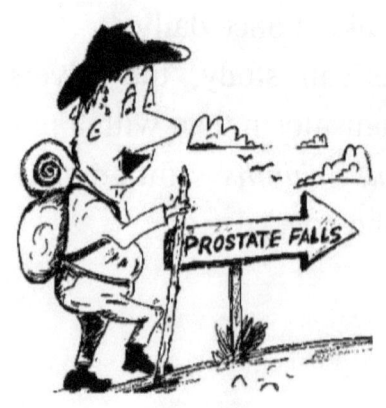

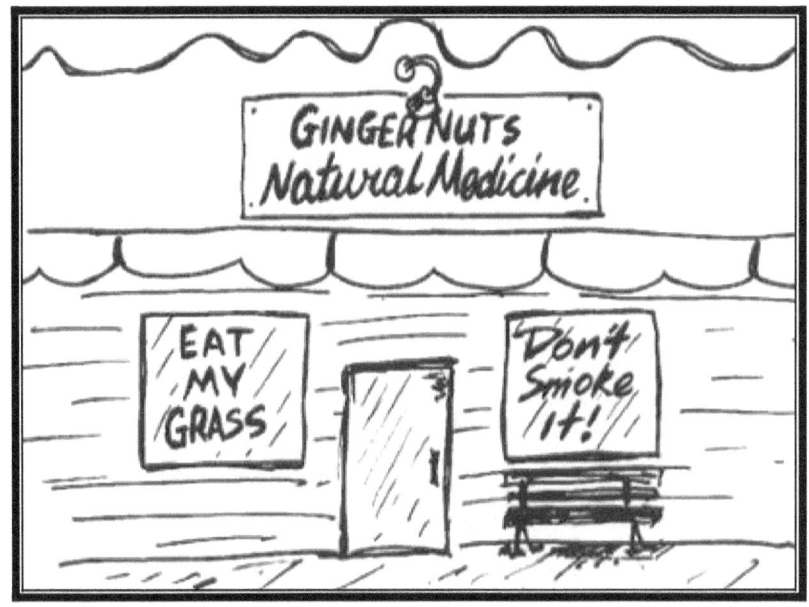

Chapter 9

Natural Methods of Prostate Treatment

Flower pollen extract, a potent and proven help in cases of prostate enlargement, comes from eight species of wildflowers that grow in the Scania district of Southern Sweden. This is not the same as bee pollen; flower pollen isn't taken and digested by bees before being processed.

The British Journal of Urology, August 1999 states *Standardised Flower Pollen Extract* is well tolerated and improves overall urological symptoms, including nocturia. *Cernitin* the major ingredient in *Cernilton flower pollen,* increases body tissue's resistance to invasion by outside agents, thus creating an anti-inflammatory effect. The other pollens work to promote urination, which is typically suppressed by prostate disorders. It has been widely used in Europe for the last 50 years to treat the symptoms of BPH and is now becoming popular in the United States and Asia as well.

Double blind tests performed by urologists at Upsala University in Sweden examined the effects of a substance on a group of BPH patients as compared against a similar group taking a harmless "placebo", or sugar pill. They found the flower pollen extract to be authentically beneficial to 90 per cent of men who take it.

Clinical studies using Cernilton show that it reduces the size and congestion of the prostate cells while urinary flow rate and clearance are improved via the action on the smooth muscle tissue that lines the urinary system.

Long term use of the substance has shown no ill effects. Even those who's prostate did not shrink under treatment reported drops in intensity of their symptoms. Seventy-six per cent of those tested reported relief from dysuria, or difficult and painful urination. Eighty-nine per cent said their urine streams had increased markedly with the flower pollen therapy.These improvements are due to the extract's contracting effect on the smooth "detrusor" muscle, which is responsible for emptying the bladder.Some of the greatest values of Cernitin may stem from elements which are for the moment still unknown to science, however many more clinical studies have been done on it, too many to be described here.

Herbal Supplements and Vitamins.

Prostatitis and BPH have been linked with deficiencies in certain nutrients in the body. Clinical trials have shown that taking the following ingredients or a combination of them have positive effects on the prostate. Taking these will help to heal and replenish the prostate gland.

When taking these health supplements made from natural ingredients, it is important to note that quality is of utmost importance. They are most effective when the manufacturing methods used to extract the nutrients are of the highest standards.

Another plus point of natural herb supplements such as these are that they are well tolerated by the body, unlike prescribed drugs which have more invasive effects. The list provided is by no means exhaustive.

Cernitin flower pollen Extract.

As previously listed in this article.

Serenoa repens.

(Saw palmetto berry extract).

Brand name – *Permixon*

.

This agent is derived from the olive-sized berries of the saw palmetto tree and is the most popular physiotherapeutic agent used in the treatment of BPH.

The exact mechanism of its action has not been confirmed, although numerous mechanisms have been proposed. These include an anti-inflammatory effect, anti-androgenic activity, inhibitory effect on type 1 and 2 isoenzymes of ruductase, and inhibition of prolactin and growth factor-induced cell proliferation. *Permixon* was studied over a three-month period and was shown to improve urine flow and reduce the symptoms of BPH.

Pygeum Africanum (African plum)

.

In traditional African medicine a tea made from powdered bark of this tall evergreen tree is used to control urinary disorders in men.

Fadenan.

Today, this supplement is commonly used in France; it is frequently sold in combination with saw palmetto and other agents as part of pills for male health. Traditionally the bark was gathered, powdered, then steeped in hot water and used as tea. Pygeum contains phytostrols, which have anti-inflammatory properties. They work to decrease prostatic swelling, reduce harmful prostaglandins that cause prostatic inflammation, and to diminish prolactin, which in turn decreases the prostates uptake of testosterone.

In one double-blind, placebo-controlled, randomised trial with 263 men in Germany, urinary symptoms improved in 66 per cent of men given the extract, compared to 31 per cent given a placebo. Although most side effects were in two instances gastrointestinal side effects were sufficient to cause men to discontinue treatment.

Stinging nettle (Urtica dioica).

There are at least 16 different preparations of this extract taken from the roots of stinging nettle. The roots contain a mixture of lectins, phenols, sterols and lignin's. Despite its widespread use in Germany for treating BPH there are limited clinical data about its efficacy for this condition. Two double-blind placebo controlled studies were conducted 10 years ago, but with few patients and in trials of less than three months, the data produced were of little value.

Beta – Sitosterol complex.

Many different herbs have been used to try and control Benign Prostate Hypertrophy (BPH) and urinary tract problems. People have used *pumpkinseeds, Red Yeast Rice, Stinging Nettle, Saw Palmetto, Rye Grass Extracts* and many others over the years to try and control these problems.

Analysing these products show they have one thing in common to control BPH and that is *Beta – Sitosterol complex.*

In Benign Prostatic Hyperlasia (BPH) Beta – sitosterol complex binds to prostatic tissue, inhibits prostaglandin synthesis in the prostate, and has anti-inflammatory activity. Independent studies have shown beta – sitosterol complex significantly improves urinary tract symptoms and *increases maximum urinary flow* and decreases *postvoid residual urine volume.* (The amount of urine left in the bladder after urinating).

Green Tea.

After water, tea is the most popular drink in the world. Green tea, called the *"froth of liquid jade"* and the *"elixir of life"* by ancient Chinese poets, is a healthful brew that you should add it to your repertoire of disease fighters and drink, at the very least two cups daily. Although black, oolong, and green teas are all made from the leaf of the plant *Camellia sinenis,* green tea is the only one of the three in which the leaves are not crushed and oxidised. Instead they are steamed, which prevents oxidation, then they are rolled and dried. Herb teas, of course, are not "true" teas at all, but some combination of the roots, leaves or flowers of plants other than Camellia sinenis.

Probably the first book to tout the benefits of green tea was written in 1211AD by the monk Eisai who called it a "miraculous medicine for the maintenance of health".

Although the Chinese have claimed for thousands of years that the tea had healthful properties, only recently have scientists been able to investigate these claims by isolating the components of tea.

Dr. Lester Mitscher, a professor of medicinal chemistry at the University of Kansas in Lawrence, advised the editors of *Bottom Line Personal* – that green tea contains the strongest known disease – fighting antioxidant. Called *epigallocatechin gallate,* or *EGCG,* it is a particular kind of *bioflavonoid* that is *25 times more effective as an antioxidant than vitamin E and 100 times more effective than vitamin C, both of which are also contained in green tea.*

Not found in black tea or only in small amounts (5 to 10 mg per cup compared to 40-90 mg per cup in green tea)

. EGCG is a member of a family of chemicals known as polyphenols, naturally occurring compounds that act as powerful antioxidants. (Bioflavonoids are a type of polyphenol). It works by interfering with or inhibiting the production of *urokinase,* an enzyme crucial for cancer growth and one of the most frequently found enzymes in human cancer. In tests conducted at the cancer prevention division of the National Cancer Research institute in Tokyo, Dr. H. Fujiki and his team of researchers were able to reduce the number of tumours in animals by 73 per cent using EGCG.

Although the effects of EGCG specifically on humans has yet to be determined, hints of its effect were evident as early as the 1970's when epidemiologists discovered that the people living in the *Shizouoka Prefecture* in central Japan had lower death rates from all forms of cancer than those living in other areas. After careful examinations of a number of factors, the only difference they could find was that the residents of *Shizouoka Prefecture,* where a lot of tea plants were grown, drank significantly more green tea than people living in areas with higher rates of cancer.

Some researchers have speculated that at least one of the reasons why Japanese become more susceptible to prostate cancer when they emigrate to the west is the decrease in their consumption of green tea. In a laboratory study where testosterone was added to prostate cancer cells to make them grow, the addition of green tea extract caused them to grow more slowly. The more green tea, the slower the growth.

Japanese researches are beginning to accumulate evidence that drinking green tea also reduces cholesterol levels, as well a lowering triglycerides, blood pressure and body fat in laboratory rats. You should be aware however that these studies use high potent amounts of green tea – the equivalent for humans of anywhere from 5 to 20 cups of green tea daily. If you don't want to consume that many cups, you can increase the benefits of each single cup by adding green tea extract.

Zinc.

For more than 50 years science has known that seminal fluid from healthy prostate gland contains a high concentration of zinc. *One ejaculation may contain nearly all the zinc absorbed by the body in one day.*

Zinc deficiency in males can have serious consequences. It can lead to infertility and in severe cases, impotency. Some evidence also shows that a lack of zinc may be the culprit in cases of chronic prostatitis. In a study at Chicago's Cook County Hospital, the zinc content of semen samples from chronic prostatitis patients was measured against samples taken from normal, healthy men.

The prostatitis sufferer's semen contained 50mgs of zinc per millilitre. The normal samples contained an average of

448mg per millilitre – more than nine times that of the prostatitis sufferers.

In another study, 200 male patients with prostatitis were given zinc supplements. With doses of 11 to 34mg per day over four months, more than 70 per cent of the men reported their symptoms disappeared.

In St Louis, a Washington University school of Medicine study indicated that zinc has antibacterial properties that may protect the prostate from infections. However, men already infected with bacterial prostatitis did not respond to zinc therapy. The US Recommended Daily Allowance for zinc is 15mg per day for adults. Although some nutritionists disagree, many doctors say it is difficult to get enough zinc from a normal diet. Shellfish are the best dietary source of zinc.

As a daily supplement, men should take no more than 30mg of zinc each day. Not all zinc taken into the body is absorbed, and too much may interfere with the body's processing of other minerals like iron and copper.

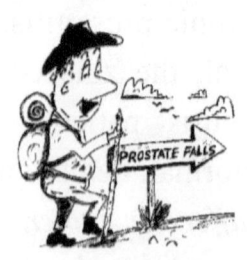

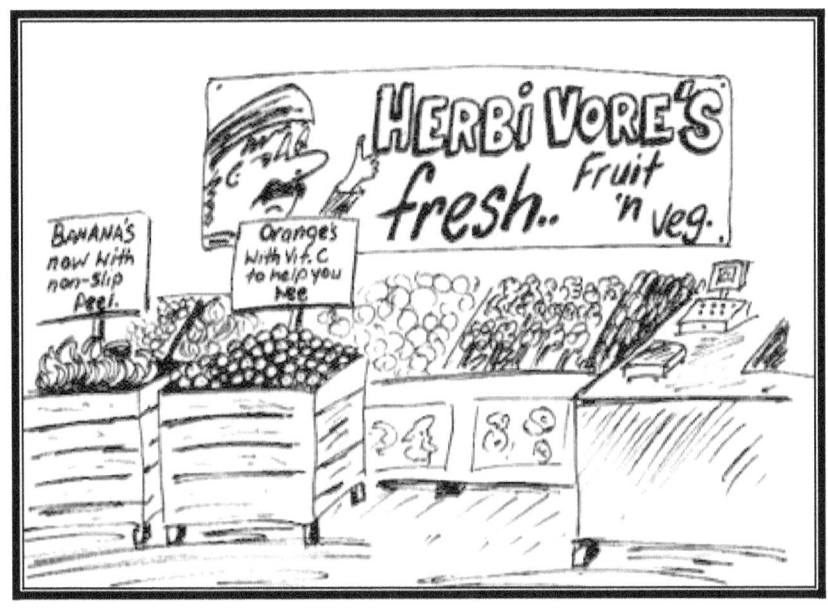

Chapter 10

Change YourDiet

Diet plays a key role in determining our overall health. It has been shown that certain types of food can trigger bodily dysfunction's including prostatitis and prostatic hypertrophy.

A significant portion of our modern diet consists of processed and artificial "junk" food. The processed toxic chemicals that the average person consumes are accumulated in the body's system all the way from childhood to adulthood. It's no wonder that we are experiencing new diseases such as heart disease, cancer, etc, at what seems like epidemic proportions. Simply put, we are what we eat; the key to good health is to eat a wholesome balanced diet.

Often it seems so much easier to just consume the processed diet that has been prepared for our convenience and then see a doctor to get a prescription for antibiotics when we fall ill. There are of course only so much drugs can do for you.

Don't wait until the doctor schedules surgery for your BPH condition before you act, it might well be too late. Almost everybody who has undergone surgery for enlarged prostate (TURP) if given the opportunity to live their life again and to choose between facing the after effects of surgery and making conscious decisions to change their diet chose the diet option.

Reduce the intake of the following.

Coffee

Tea (black)

Refined sugar

Artificial sweeteners

Preservatives

Salt

Alcohol

Most doctors agree that men with prostate problems may want to avoid certain types of food that interfere with medications, irritate swollen tissues, promote urination are linked with androgen, cholesterol or carcinogen production.

Meat preserved with nitrites – like bacon, cold cuts, and sausage or smoked chops – should be avoided. Nitrites are carcinogens (cancer linked to chemicals) and are known to irritate enlarged glands.

Other items to avoid include chocolate, caffeine, pickled foods, margarine and processed foods. Alcohol is very irritating to prostate tissue, and some men react to flavourings in certain drinks with a type of chronic prostatitis.

Improve your selenium intake.

Selenium is an essential trace element discovered in 1817 by Swedish chemist Jons Jakob Berzelius, who named it after the moon goddess Selene. Selenium originates in the soil, where it is absorbed by growing plants. Almost half of a man's supply of selenium is concentrated in the testicles and portions of the seminal ducts adjacent to the prostate gland. A strong association between a low selenium level and the risk of developing gastrointestinal and prostatic cancers was established in a 1983 study.

Good Sources of Selenium

Whole grain products

Garlic

Onions

Shellfish

Meat

Chicken

Mushrooms

Milk

Supplements are not recommended, as there is only a narrow margin between safe and toxic doses of selenium.

Eat a low fat diet.

Maintaining a low fat diet is one of the simplest things you can do for your general health, for the health of your prostate, and for giving your immune system a hearty boost.

Select lean meats and low fat products.

Chicken

Seafood

Eggs

Low-fat dairy products

Skim milk

Unsaturated fats (olive and canola oils)

Avoid fat filled salad dressings and rich and spicy sauces. Bake or broil foods instead of frying.

Consume more soy-based foods.

Japanese and Chinese men have another diet advantage over men from other cultures. They consume a lot of food made from soybeans, such as miso soup, tofu (also known as "bean curd"), and products made from it.

Because tofu is soft and porous, it will easily absorb the flavour of any dish in which it is cooked. Tofu is an excellent protein. In the United States, soymilk has become an important food for some health-minded people, and especially for those who don't like milk or don't digest well. Soy-based foods are high in phytochemicals and a substance called genisten, which some health food orientated people believe helps detoxify DHT.

Genisten has estrogen-like properties, which may inhibit the growth of prostate cancer early in its development.

Eat More Salads, Fresh Vegetables and Fruits.

Many of us have been conditioned from childhood to believe that a diet rich in animal protein is healthful and hearty. *Wrong!* Yet there are still men who will tell you proudly, "I'm a meat and potatoes man". The truth is that too much protein weakens the heart, speeds the deposits of fatty plaque in the arteries, reduces the effectiveness of the immune system, and promotes the formation of free radicals. Some nutrition experts believe that people who eat a low-protein diet generate more body heat, which means less body fat. The traditional Chinese diet contains about one-third less protein than Americans eat.

To reduce the amount of protein in your diet, *fill up on vegetables and fruits by including five to eight servings a day.* Fruits and vegetables contain *phytochemicals* (trace substances that protect plants) which are powerful *antioxidants.*

Phytochemicals help to lower cholesterol, reduce blood pressure, detoxify blood, rebuild the liver, relieve the inflammation caused by allergies and arthritis alleviates depression and impotency and helps detect and deter tumours.

Happily, for a varied diet, there are tens of thousands of them found in fruits, vegetables, beans and natural grains. One study of 122,261 men found a lower death rate from prostate cancer in men who ate green and yellow vegetables every day.

Beta-carotenes are the natural pigments that create the colour in dark green (broccoli and spinach) orange (carrots, sweet potatoes and pumpkin) red (red peppers and tomatoes) and deep-yellow vegetables and fruits (apricots, rock melons, mangoes, peaches, cabbage, winter squash and Brussel sprouts).

Converted to Vitamin A in the body, beta-carotenes repair damaged DNA, protect the mucous membranes of the mouth, nose, oesophagus and lungs (our first line of defence against invading organisms) and cell membranes and enrich and support the overall immune system.

They are one of our major sources of carotenoids, some of the most potent plant antioxidants.

Taken in general, carotenoids are a group of several kinds of pigments in fruits and vegetables and include alpha-carotene, beta-carotene, lycopene, lutein and many other compounds that are associated with a reduced cancer risk when consumed in natural foods.

Add plenty of cruciferous vegetables (Brussel sprouts, cabbage, broccoli, cauliflower and other members of the cabbage family) to your diet, as they contain dithiothiones substances that eliminate the destructive properties of cancer-causing agents.

Broccoli and Brussel sprouts, carrots and green onions also contain a potent cancer-fighting chemical called sulforaphane. Research suggests that many men who develop BPH are not consuming enough cruciferous vegetables. The irregular consumption of green and yellow vegetables was found to be significantly higher in 100 men with BPH when compared to 100 men not having BPH, hinting that these vegetables may have beneficial, prophylactic effects.

Laboratory studies have linked Vitamin A deficiency to development of different kinds of tumours, and been able to decrease prostate cancer with Vitamin A supplements.

The recommended Daily Allowance of Vitamin A is 5,000 International Units. At the most do not take more than 10,000 I.U. per day from all sources (diet plus supplements). An overdose can cause liver damage, lack of appetite, dry skin, hair loss, joint pain, irritability and headaches. Because the body does not convert beta-carotene to Vitamin A, when

Vitamin A levels are within normal ranges, eating fruits and vegetables containing beta-carotene will not lead to Vitamin A toxicity.

Cooked Tomatoes.

Lycopenes, which are found in tomatoes and given their red colour, act as a strong antioxidant and protection against lung, colon, bladder, pancreas and prostate tumours, as well as cutting heart attack risk.

In order to help reduce an enlarging prostate, the tomatoes must be cooked because lycopene is most easily absorbed when tomatoes and tomato products are cooked, especially in a little oil; they also need to be eaten at least five times a week. Could this be why Italian and Greek men have fewer prostate problems than men do in other countries? Best sources of cooked tomatoes are tomato sauce, canned tomatoes, tomato paste and tomato juice.

Garlic.

Throughout the history of humans, many cultures have used herbs not only for nutrients but also for health benefits. Garlic is one of the most medicinal of all culinary herbs. Its remains have been found in caves used by early man as long as 10,000 years ago.

The first garlic prescription was found chiselled in cuneiform on a Sumerian clay tablet dating back 3,000 years BC. The Egyptians used garlic to provide strength and nourishment to the slaves constructing the pyramids.

Garlic healing qualities have been related to various sulphur compounds it contains (although there are some 75 more), which are the key to its antibiotic and antifungal action (penicillin is also a sulphur compound). Two have received much attention, the first; alliin has neither smell nor taste nor medicinal effects. So what good is it? Well, when garlic is crushed, cut or otherwise bruised, alliin makes contact with a catalytic enzyme called alliance, which converts the alliin into allicin. A compound that is not only responsible for garlic's characteristic odour, but many of its potent health benefits.

Unfortunately, if left to stand in the air or when cooked, allicin is destroyed. The sulphur compounds in raw garlic help prevent the liver from generating too much cholesterol, help thin the blood and reduce clotting, inhibit inflammation, protect against the effect of radiation, offer antioxidant protection to cell membranes, and may provide a normalising effect on the prostate.

Garlic and its cousins (onions, shallots, leeks and chives) inhibit the production of certain enzymes (Lipoxygenase and cyclooxygenase), thus slowing the production of prostaglandin's, which are involved in the process of inflammation.

Many cancers are prostaglandin dependent, which may explain, at least in part, the anti-tumour properties of the oils of the alliin family. They also lower cholesterol, triglycerides and low-density lipoprotein (also known as LDL or bad cholesterol) levels while increasing levels of the beneficial high-density lipoprotein or HDL.

Although many nutritionists recommend garlic raw or cooked, uncrushed garlic buds (about one clove) or dried garlic at the rate of one gram per day will have beneficial effects.

The Effects of Fibre in a good Diet.

Dietary fibre refers to a wide range of plant carbohydrates that are not digested by humans. It can be divided into two types, *"soluble"* (oat bran) and *"insoluble"* (wheat bran) fibre, with the latter being thought to help reduce the risk of colorectal cancer, *fibre speeds the passage of faecal matter through the intestines, thus reducing the time the body is exposed to toxins.*

Soluble fibre also helps reduce circulating total cholesterol concentrations. Researchers have found that increasing dietary wheat bran by 10 per cent caused a 65 per cent reduction in prostate enlargement.

Good sources of fibre include beans, vegetables, whole grains and fruits. Rice, another staple in the Asian diet, is an ideal carbohydrate. It has fewer calories and is more filling than bread. Soybean fibre reduces fat levels in the blood; seaweed contains certain gums that slow fat absorption, as well as providing calcium.

Caffeine Alcohol and Spicy Foods.

Most urologists believe that caffeine (a known diuretic) alcohol and spicy foods can irritate an already enlarged prostate and suggest that you eliminate them or at least cut back on their use. They can also exacerbate bladder irritation and cause bladder spasms, which in turn, can cause reflux of urine into the prostatic ducts and contribute to symptoms of nonbacterial prostatitis.

Avoid Decongestants and Antihistamine.

Learn to read the fine print. *The most popular decongestants and antihistamines should carry warnings not to use them if a person has an enlarged prostate or BPH.* They are notorious for provoking the prostate, causing it to contract, which of course decreases urine flow. This is why for persons who need to use decongestants and antihistamines, using *Cernitin* to reduce the prostate size is an important choice. *Refer to chapter on Natural Methods of Prostate Treatment.*

Parkinson's disease medication may also cause difficulties. *Before you take over-the-counter drugs, or for that matter, any prescribed medication, check with your doctor or pharmacist if you are not sure what their effect is on the prostate.*

Smoking is a Health Hazard.

There is some evidence that cigarette smoking may indirectly affect the size of the enlarging prostate. The association between cigarette smoking and prostatic volume was investigated in 68 men with BPH by assessing changes in serum levels of four specific androgens. One of the androgens, oestradiol, showed significantly higher levels for smokers than non-smokers. Cigarette smoke is high in cadmium, a toxic heavy metal, which is markedly higher in the cancerous prostate.

There have also been reports, largely anecdotal, of positive association between smoking and prostate cancer. However, a study of 1,097 prostate cancer cases and 3,250 matched controls admitted between 1969 and 1991 to U.S. hospitals found no association between prostate cancer and former and current smoking, age started smoking, number of years smoking, cigarettes per day smoked, number of years since quitting, and lifetime tar exposure. This is not to say that smoking is not related to other types of cancers.

You've seen in this chapter that what you put into your body can actually strengthen (or weaken) your immune system, and can help fortify you against getting prostate cancer, as well as heart disease, stroke and other major killer disease.

Your body needs many nutrients to continue functioning in top form. A diet designed to promote prostate health and prevent prostate cancer is also a healthy diet. It entails a variety of foods, especially those that contain antioxidants and requires you to keep your weight under control.

Any kind of change, especially one that involves your daily eating habits, can feel stressful and uncomfortable at first. So, as you choose more foods high in nutrients (such as vegetables, grains and fresh fruit) think of this new regime as strengthening your immune system. Some determination and self-control may be required, but your immune system will love you for it.

Cernitin for Prostate health and to reduce symptoms of BPH.

Cernitin of course, is at the heart of the *man's natural treatment*. For maximum effectiveness it is recommended you take at least two 63 mg Cernitin tablets twice a day. This is the amount that has been used in all clinical studies, and it seems to be the most effective at treating the symptoms of BPH.

Cernitin has proven its effectiveness again and again in research studies. It is a safe and natural supplement that provides relief to many men suffering from the annoying symptoms of BPH. Significantly, it is without the drawbacks of many treatments, the invasiveness, danger and recovery from surgery and the negative side of many prescription drugs.

Change of life style—could be the go
Exercise and diet---may help with the flow
A rebore of Willie---is not much fun
But he will work better---after it's done.

Willie Tinkle's Food Guide for Prostate and Sexual Health.

Zinc, found in seminal fluid. Zinc deficiency
can lead to infertility and impotence.

Found in Shellfish are the best source of dietary
Zinc.

Selenium, Found in the testicles. Low level can lead to
the risk of developing gastrointestinal and prostate cancer.

Found in: Whole grain products
Onions
Shellfish
Lean meat
Chicken
Mushrooms

Milk
Garlic

Soy based foods:

Contain Phytochemicals and Genisten.

Genisten has Estrogen- like properties which may help inhibit the early growth of prostate cancer.

Found in:
Soy milk
Miso soup
Tofu (bean curd)
Soy bread
Food made from soybeans

Lycopene's: A strong antioxidant.

Found in: Cooked tomatoes

Beta carotenes: Exists in the colouring of fruit
And vegetables. Repairs damaged DNA.

Found in:
 Broccoli, spinach
Carrots, sweet potato pumpkin
Red peppers and tomatoes
Apricots, rock melons,
Mangoes, peaches.

Dithiothiones: Have cancer-fighting properties

Sulforaphane:

Found in:
Broccoli, Brussels sprout, carrots,

Green onions, cabbage, cauliflower
And any member of the cabbage family.

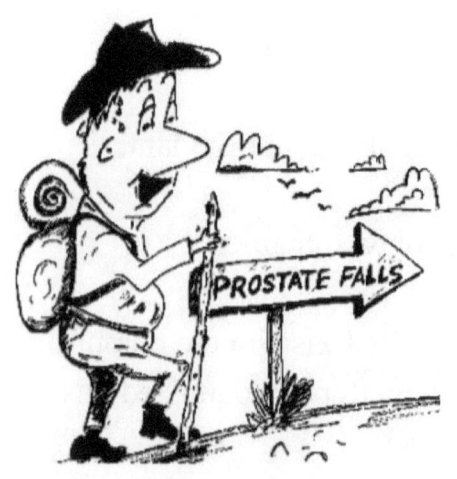

Willie Tinkle's **Diet to Good Health.**

Foods allowed freely – use as desired.
All vegetables not listed as bread choices.

Low fat milk	diet cordial	diet soft drink
Diet jelly	junket tablets	low joule
Dressing		

Plain gelatine	rhubarb	soda water
Natural bran	unsweet pickles	bonox
Herbs	passionfruit	bovrill
Spices	lemons	mineral water
Soy sauce	lemon juice	essence
Vinegar	Marmite	Promite
Vegemite	Worcestershire	
Fish paste	sauce	

Foods to Avoid.

Sugar	honey	syrups
Lollies	jams'	marmalade
Cakes	sweets	sweet biscuits
Ice cream	nuts	pastries
Desserts	icy poles	chocolates
Cordial	soft drinks	condensed milk
Dried fruit	sweetened fruit	health bars
Chewing gum	thickening	fatty meats
Chips	pate & dips	salami
Frankfurt's	corn/wheat flour	fried foods
Black tea	coffee & alcohol	sweetened
Fruit juice		

Preparing Your Food

SOUP   Make stock the day before, cool
And remove fat.

Suitable vegetables as desired
Use barley, rice, noodles, dried beans
200mls in soup = 1 serve bread
Commercial soup made with water
200mls = 1 serve bread.

MEAT   Use lean cuts (rump, fillet, round)
Remove visible fat before cooking
Don't add fat or oil.
Grill Don't Fry, roast on rack
Or BBQ
When cooking stews or casseroles,
Allow to cool and remove fat.

POULTRY   Steam, boil or roast, remove the
Skin.

FISH   Steam, poach, grill or bake in foil
One teaspoon of oil may be used to
Cook non-oily white fleshed fish.

EGGS   Boiled, poached, scrambled,
Omelette.

VEGETABLES   Steam, boil, microwave, dry
Bake.
Bake in oven wrapped in foil

Flavour with herbs and spices
Don't overcook. No added oil

DESSERTS

Stew fruit with spices
 (Cinnamon, nutmeg, cloves and mixed spice)
Set stewed or tinned fruit in Low calorie jelly
plain Gelatine.
 Whip low cal jelly for a different texture
Use plain yoghurt as part of your milk allowance.

David Eames

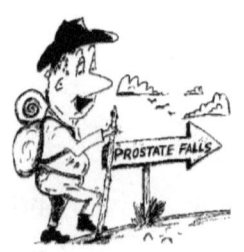

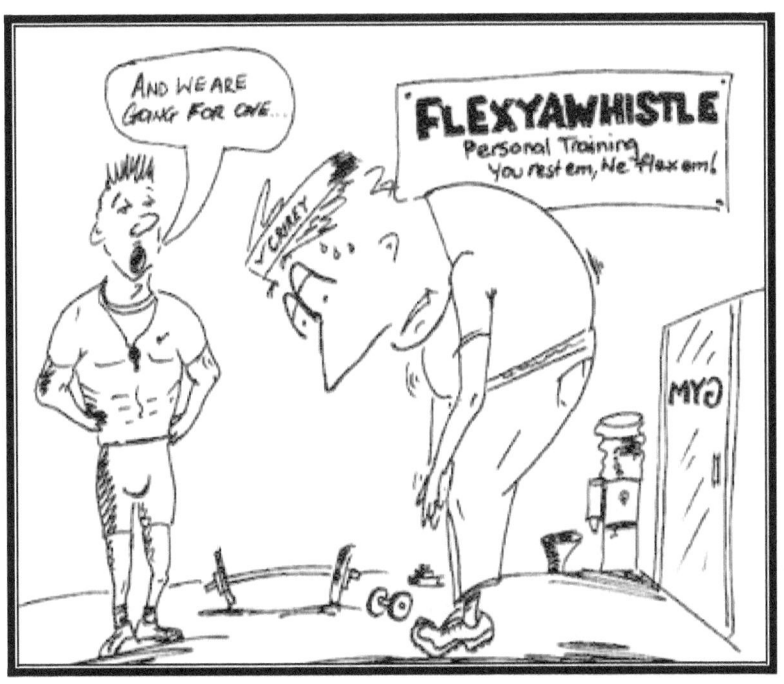

Chapter 11

Exercise

Exercise has so many health benefits that it's hard to keep track of them all. Although there are no specific exercise programs that can prevent BPH, we do know that if you are exercising, you are increasing your overall general health and boosting your immune system. Regular exercise makes it easier to fight off all kinds of health problems, including prostate problems.

Exercise burns calories, helping to control weight. It lowers the risk of heart disease and cancer and boosts strength no matter what your age while reducing your cholesterol level and keeping your bones strong and flexible. It also helps to reverse the lowered basal metabolic rate that most people think comes naturally with ageing. It is in fact almost wholly caused by loss of muscle mass which is also reversed by exercise.

Most fitness experts consider fitness as involving the key components of aerobic endurance, muscular strength, muscular endurance, flexibility, and body composition. A good fitness program strives to attain balance between them all.

Aerobic endurance is the ability to exercise whole muscle groups over an extended period of time at moderate intensity.

Muscular strength is of course the capacity of your body's muscles to exert a certain amount of force, while *muscular endurance* refers to how well your muscles can maintain or repeatedly generate that force.

Flexibility, being able to stretch your muscles and the tendons and ligaments that connect muscles to your bones decreases the risk of injury while exercising.

Body composition is concerned with the relationship of fat, bone and muscle in your body. Their ratio provides an overall view of your health and fitness level.

To develop the best level of fitness for you, start off moderately. As you progress, work your way *gradually* into a routine that suits you.

Slow graduations not only ease your body into exercise and the demands you make on it, but they help you to avoid injury. Contrary to popular myth, running is not the best exercise to get fit, because there is no one "best" exercise.

Don't keep up the same old routine over and over if it's boring for you. Have some fun. One of the quickest ways to avoid exercising is to develop a workout that bores you. Adding new exercises to your workout, or changing activities, can break the monotony and add interest to your routine.

Stagger the intensity of your workouts and alternate by days the type of exercise you do. Leave at least one day between muscle-building exercises. Rest and alternating workouts allow your body time to recover and grow, help build endurance, and prevent injury.

Don't dehydrate yourself while exercising, during exercise; the body needs water to replace water loss.

If you become thirsty during a workout, you have already passed out of a "safe" stage of hydration, take fluids immediately. Avoid caffeine or alcohol when exercising as both can cause dehydration.

Try exercising in the morning. It is the best time of the day to exercise. You're usually more rested in the am. so you will get a better workout. You'll be energised for the rest of the day, ready to take on the challenges.

Simple Rules for Any Exercise Method.

Don't eat for two hours before vigorous exercise.
Drink plenty of fluids before, during and after your workout.
Adjust activity according to the weather and reduce it when fatigued or ill.
When exercising, listen to the body's warning symptoms, and consult a physician if exercise induces chest pain, irregular heartbeat, undue fatigue, nausea, unexpected breathlessness or light- headedness.

Warming up.

Warm up exercises should be practised for 5 to 10 minutes at the beginning of an exercise session. Older people need a longer period to warm up their muscles.
Low-level aerobic exercise is the best approach, such as walking briskly, swinging the arms or jogging in place.

Cooling down.

To cool down, one should walk slowly until the heart rate is 10 to 15 beats above resting rate. Stopping too suddenly can sharply reduce blood pressure, a danger for older people, and may cause muscle cramping.

Stretching may be appropriate for the cooling down period, but it must be done carefully for warming up because it can injure cold muscles.
Aerobic (Endurance) Training.

Regular aerobic exercise:

Builds endurance. Keeps the heart pumping at a steady and elevated rate for an extended period, boosts HDL (the "good") cholesterol levels and helps control blood pressure.
Strengthens the bones and spine.
Helps maintain normal weight.

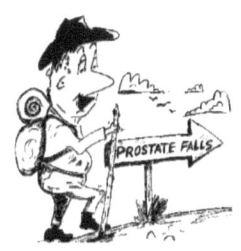

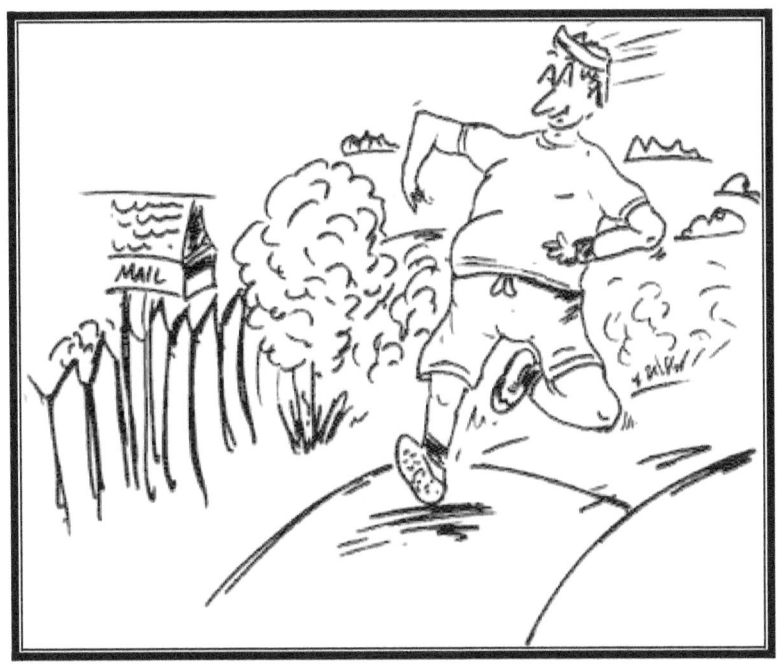

Types of Aerobic Exercise.

Low to moderate impact exercises: Walking, swimming, stair climbing, step classes, rowing and bicycle riding.
Nearly anyone in reasonable health can engage in some low to moderate – impact exercise.

Brisk walking burns as many calories as jogging for the same distance and poses less risk for injury to muscle and bone.

High - Impact Exercises:

Running, dance exercises, tennis, racquetball and squash.

High-impact exercises should be performed no more than every other day and less for those who are overweight, elderly, out of condition or have an injury or other medical problem that would preclude high-impact.

Aerobic programs:

As little as one hour per week of aerobic exercises is helpful, but three to four hours per week are optimal. Some research indicates that simply walking briskly for three or more hours per week reduces the risk for coronary heart disease by 65%. In general, the following guidelines are useful for most individuals.

People who are out of shape or elderly should start aerobic training gradually. For example, they may start with 5 to 10 minutes of low – impact aerobic activity every other day and build toward a goal of 30 minutes a day, three to seven times per week. (For heart protection, frequency of exercises may be more important than duration).

Swimming is an ideal exercise for many elderly and certain people with physical limitations including individuals with muscle, joint, or bone problems and those who suffer from exercise-induced asthma.

People who seek to lose weight should aim for six to seven low – impact workouts per week. One way of gauging the optimal intensity of exercise is to aim for a *"talking pace" which is enough to work up a sweat and still be able to converse with a friend without gasping for breath.* As fitness increases, the talking pace will become faster and faster.

Heart Rate Goal.

Heart rate is the standard guide for determining aerobic exercise intensity. It can be determined by counting one's own pulse or with the use of a heart rate monitor. Exercise does not increase the maximum heart rate. It strengthens the heart so that it can pump more blood at this maximum level and can sustain this level longer with less strain.

Attaining target heart rate is not the key to the health benefits of physical activity, exercising at a steady pace is the first goal.

To determine one's own maximum heart rate per minute simply subtract one's age from 220.

To Determine Heart Rate:

Measure the pulse by pressing the first two fingers of one hand gently on either the artery on the inside of the wrist or on a carotid artery. This artery is located under the jaw either on the right or left side of the neck. Count pulse beats for 10 seconds.

Multiply the results by six. This gives the per-minute total.

The following are general goals for adults:

Most healthy adults should aim for a heart rate of about 60% to 85% of its maximum rate during actual exercise.

People who have been sedentary should first aim for 50% to 60% of maximum heart rate.

People with heart risk factor (e.g. Hypertension, high cholesterol levels, diabetes or obesity) should aim for 55% to 75%.

Target Heart Rate for a One-Minute Pulse Count.

Age.	Low. 60% max.	High. 85% max.
20	120	170
30	114	162
40	108	153
50	102	145
60 +	96	136

Strength or Resistance Training.

Benefits of Strength Exercise.
While aerobic exercise increases endurance and helps the heart, it does not build upper body strength or tone muscles. Strength training exercises provide the following benefits:

Builds muscle strength while burning fat.
Helps maintain bone density.
Improves digestion.

It is also associated with a lower risk for heart disease, possibly because it lowers LDL (the so called "bad") cholesterol levels.

Strength exercise is beneficial for everyone, even people in their 90's. It is the only form of exercise that can slow and even reverse the decline in muscle mass, bone density and strength that occurs with ageing.
(Please note: people at risk for cardiovascular disease should not perform strength exercises without consulting your physician).

Types of Muscle Contractions.

Isometric contractions-There is no change in the length of the muscle. For example, pushing against the wall.

Concentric contractions-These movements shorten muscles (for example the "up" phase of when the biceps curl up while lifting weights). Eccentric contractions-These movements lengthen muscles, (the "down" phase as weights are lowered).

Strength Training Regimens.

Strength training involves intense and short duration activities. *For beginners, adding 10 to 20 minutes of modest strength training two to three times per week may be appropriate.*

The following are some guidelines for starting a strength regime:

The sequence of a strength training session should begin with training large muscles and multiple joints at higher intensity and end with small muscles and single joint exercises at lower intensities.

Both concentric (shortening) and eccentric (lengthening) muscle actions should be performed.

Emphasising eccentric contractions (the movement that lengthens muscles) *is of increasing interest. This approach involves slowing and increasing the duration of these "down" movements. It appears to significantly increase blood flow, and some evidence suggests it may achieve stronger muscles more quickly and improve cardiovascular functions compared to standard movements. It may be particularly beneficial for older people and some people with chronic health problems.*

Eccentric training increases the risk of muscle soreness and injury, however, and this approach is still controversial.
Strength training involves repetitious, i.e., moving specific muscles in the same pattern against a resisting force (such as a weight) for a pre-set number of times.

First choose a weight that is about half of what would require a maximum effort in one repetition. In other words, if it would take maximum effort to do a single repetition with an 8kg weight then the person would start with a 4kg weight. In the beginning, most people can start with one set of 8 to 15 repetitions per muscle group with low weights. As individuals are able to perform one or two repetitions over their set routine weights can be increased by 2% to 10%.

Breathe slowly and rhythmically. Exhale as the movement begins, inhale as the movement ends.

The first half of each repetition typically lasts two to three seconds. The return to the original position lasts four seconds.

An alternative technique called "super slow" training stretches out one repetition to a 14 second count. This method places far more stress on the muscle group, so fewer repetitions are needed. A full week recovery is required before repeating this workout. The goal is to initiate changes in the muscles so that the body continues to burn calories after the exercise. Some people report dramatic results from this approach, but scientific verification is not available. It is very tedious in any case and people have a hard time sticking to it. People with high blood pressure should not use this approach. Joints should be moved rhythmically through their full range of motion during a repetition and not locked up. For maximum benefit, one should allow 48 hours between workouts for full muscle recovery.

To Summarise.

At least half the age-related changes to the body's muscles, bones and joints are caused by disuse. Recent studies show that less than one in 10 Australians over the age of 50 years does enough exercise to improve or maintain cardiovascular fitness.

Walking is an excellent form of exercise for people of all ages and abilities. Prepare for a walk by warming up; wear comfortable clothes and shoes. Drink lots of water.

Cold joints, tendons and muscles are more likely to get strained or sprained by sudden movement or exertion.

Concentrate on warming up the specific muscle groups you will be using in your exercise and include stretches.

Strength training assumes even more importance as one age's. One 2000 study found that men between the ages of 60 and 75 have the same potential to gain strength as men in their 20's. As little as one day a week of resistance training improves overall strength and agility.

Flexibility exercises promote healthy muscle growth and help to reduce the stiffness and loss of balance that accompanies ageing. People with a chronic illness should consult a doctor before choosing any exercise programme.

At least 30 minutes a day of moderate intensity physical activity on most days are considered the minimum amount of exercise. A brisk walk is a good example.

Be active every day in as many ways as you can. Walk or cycle instead of using the car, do things for your self instead of using labour saving devices.

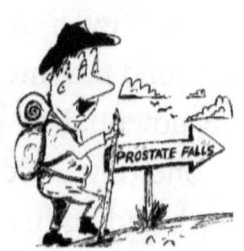

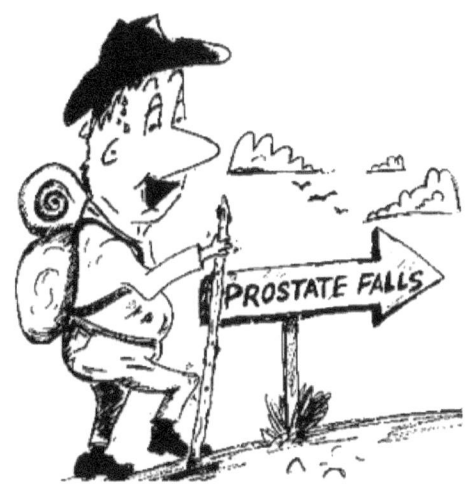

Chapter 12

Prostate Symptoms Quiz

You may feel embarrassed to talk to your doctor about urinary problems. Like grey and thinning hair, such problems are part of ageing.

One of the causes of urinary symptoms of men over fifty is a treatable condition called benign prostatic hyperplasia (BPH). In fact, it has been estimated by age sixty; one in every four males will require treatment of their urinary symptoms caused by BPH. Taking this quiz will help you and your doctor decide whether you could benefit from BPH treatment.

If you have experienced one or more of the following symptoms in the previous month, please consult your medical professional.

Incomplete emptying

Have you had the sensation of not emptying your bladder completely after you have finished urinating?

Frequency

Have you had to urinate again less than two hours after you finished urinating?

Intermittency

Have you found you stopped and started again several times when you urinated?

Urgency

Have you found it difficult to postpone urination?

Weak stream

Have you had a weak urinary stream?

Straining

Have you had to push or strain to begin urination?

Nocturia

How many times did you most typically get up to urinate from the time you went to bed at night until the time you got up in the morning?

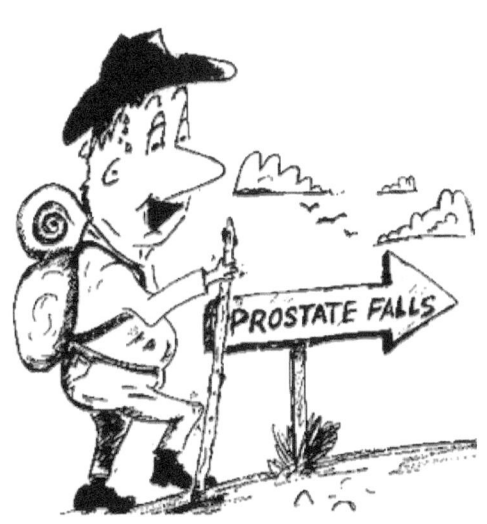

David Eames

Chapter13

FLOW TEST.

Requires:
1 – Measuring utensil marked up to at least 300mls.
1 – Watch with second hand.

Start with full bladder.

When stream becomes full, urinate into your measuring cup for 10 seconds, and then move the cup away.

Normal urine flow is 20mls per second.

After a 10 second test your utensil should hold at least 200mls.

If your test yields noticeably less consult your doctor.

A Picture is better than a Thousand Words.

Sweet Dreams *Willie.*

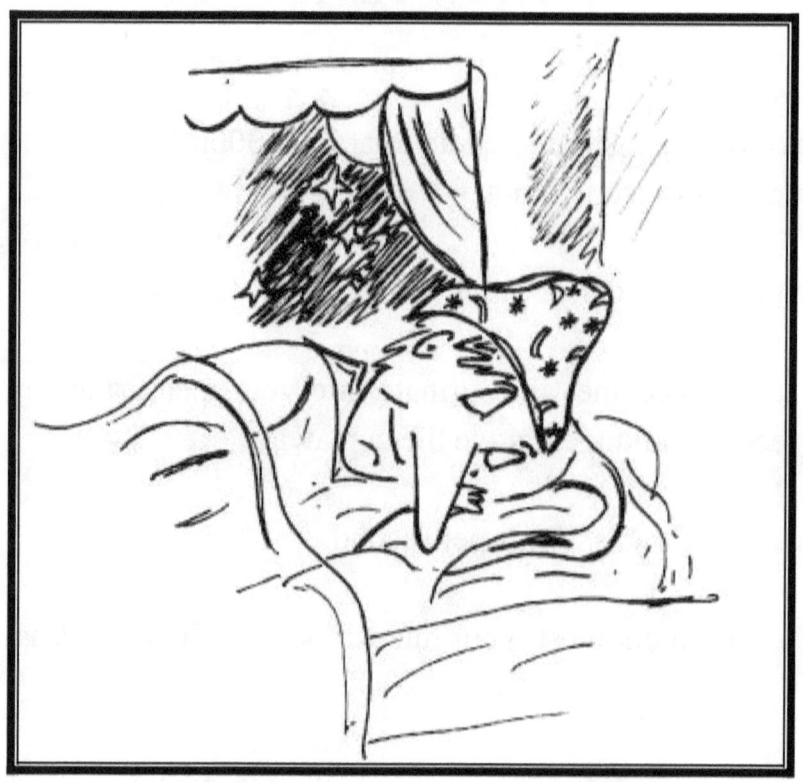

Willie Tinkle

David Eames

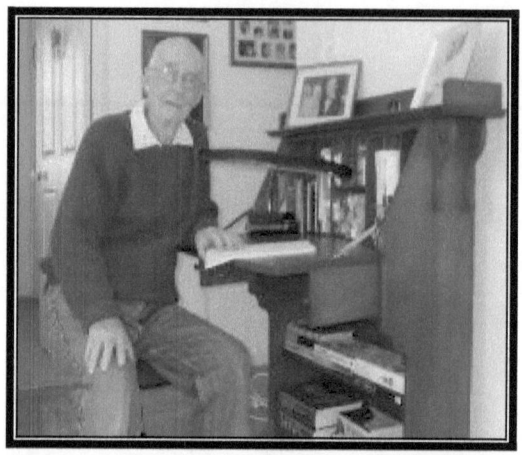

About the Author

David's parents were travelling Showmen travelling extensively within the eastern states of Australia. He was born on the road during the Great Depression.

When World War Two began he had the opportunity to attend a tiny bush School of twelve Pupils. As sixth grade was as far as he could go at the bush School, he could sit at the rear of the class and study Diesel Engineering, graduating with a certificate at age fifteen.

Always interested in engineering design he designed and built a house with the appearance of a spaceship, and as a result of its aerodynamic shape would withstand cyclonic winds from all points of the compass.

One of his designs was displayed at the Sydney Olympics in the Australian Technology Showcase which had a limit of 200 Australian Products.

He is the author of **The Showie Boy**, an Autobiaography of his life growing up on the **Showground**s of Australia during **The Great Depression**. He is a singer/songwriter, plays the Ukulele and the Didgeridoo. As a member of the Queensland Writers Centre, he is the author of several short stories.

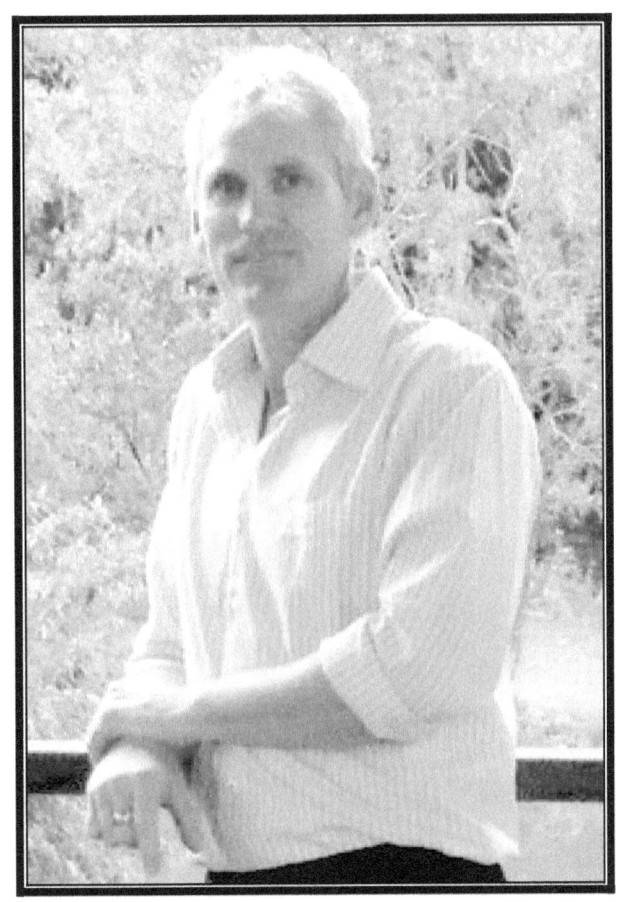

Cover design and illustrator
Artist-Phillip D Eames